# TEENAGE PREGNANCY

## A GLOBAL TRAGEDY

How you can understand the tragedy
of children having children.

SUCCESS OMA

# DEDICATION

This book is dedicated to all teenagers/teenage Mom, mothers, fathers and guidance.

# CONTENTS

# INTRODUCTION

Teen pregnancy can be characterized as pregnancy that happens in little kids underneath the age of twenty, whether or not they are hitched or of grown-up age. Young pregnancy has been expanding at a disturbing rate particularly in Africa, United States, Asia, Europe and others.

It has turned into a worldwide concern since it influences the youngster and her family, yet the general public overall. An Expansion in young pregnancy will eventually lead to expanded kid destitution as well as the kid's prosperity.

# TEENS PREGNANCY

Teen pregnancy is the point at which a lady under 20 gets pregnant. It generally alludes to youngsters between the ages of 15-19. Yet, it can incorporate young ladies as youthful as 10. It's likewise called youngster pregnancy or juvenile pregnancy
High schooler pregnancy has been called a pandemic. Notwithstanding, the heartbreaking extents of this issue are best seen when the effect of a pregnancy upon one terrified teen young lady is thought of. In any event, she will encounter extraordinary changes in her day to day existence that will profoundly affect herself as well as her family and friends and family.
It would be oversimplified to believe high schooler pregnancy to be simply an issue

of contraception. The proof demonstrates that high schooler pregnancy includes various complex social and intense subject matters.

## Contributing Elements

Research shows that numerous high schooler moms come from broken homes. My entire life all I have at any point needed was a genuine family, is the repetitive cry of numerous pregnant teenagers. Clearly, then, useless families might make way for adolescent pregnancy. An effort program that helps high schooler moms found that they frequently have unstable associations with their moms and no associations with their dads. Anita, who became a mother at 18 years old, recalls that despite the fact that her single parent endeavored to accommodate her tangibly, Mirabella actually felt the close to home void made by the shortfall of her dad.

Different young ladies become unwed moms as an immediate consequence of assault. For some of them, the injury appears to set off profound agony that might manifest later in a disastrous direction.

Jenny, for instance, was assaulted at age 15. After that, she recalls that she became pointless. At the point when I was 19, I got pregnant. Sexual maltreatment may likewise set off sensations of uselessness, I never felt deserving of anything, mourns Jenny.

Mirabella went through a comparative experience between the ages of 7 and 11, she was attacked by a young person.

She couldn't stand it, and she was accusing herself.

She became pregnant at 17 years old. Then again, a few young people are the survivors of their own carelessness and interest.

A few young people apparently don't get a handle on the association among sex and pregnancy. In one overview, adolescent moms frequently announced being stunned or shocked to find they were pregnant regardless of whether they had not been utilizing contraception.

In any case, the changing mentalities toward sex have had the greatest impact on adolescent pregnancy. We live in times when individuals are admirers of joys as opposed to admirers of God 2 Timothy 3:1-4

Having a child without both mom and dad present, youngsters may never again convey the very disgrace that it did in times past. Why, in certain areas youngsters might try and view having a child as a prize or superficial point of interest of some kind.

## Profound Fallout.

The real factors of adolescent parenthood are very not quite the same as energetic dreams. After discovering that they are pregnant, young ladies frequently experience a tempest of feelings. Many concede feeling stunned or dazed. Normal responses incorporate indignation, culpability, and disavowal, says the American Institute of Kid and Juvenile Psychiatry. Refusal can be hazardous, however, as it might keep a young lady from seeking after required clinical treatment.

I got frightened, and reviewed Evelyn existing apart from everything else she encountered the aftereffects of her experience with sex. Numerous pregnant young ladies don't have somebody to trust in or are too embarrassed to even consider discussing what is going on. As anyone might expect, then, some become overpowered by responsibility and dread. Numerous pregnant teenagers likewise experience extreme discouragement. I couldn't have cared less about living, and I couldn't have cared less if I kicked the bucket, say Jenny.

Anyway a little kid might respond at first, she should ultimately settle on various extensive choices for her as well as her youngster.

# THE PROBLEM/SOLUTIONS OF TEENS PREGNANCY:

The issues related with adolescent pregnancy as featured by Guttmacher Organization
1999 are as recorded underneath:
 There is a higher gamble that children brought into the world from young moms are conceived too soon, or that
they have a low weight upon entering the world.
 The moms may likewise experience

confusions or hardships upon entering the world; they have a
higher gamble of pallor than moms matured 20-24.

 A pregnancy is best trailed via prepared clinical staff during its course. Adolescent moms are more averse to get pre-birth care, frequently looking for it in the third trimester, if
by any means. The Guttmacher Foundation reports that 33% of pregnant youngsters get
inadequate pre-birth care and that their youngsters are bound to experience the ill effects of wellbeing
issues in adolescence or be hospitalized than those brought into the world to more seasoned ladies.

 Like most different young people, teen moms might experience the ill effects of unfortunate sustenance. This may
lead to them having explicit diseases

connected with awful nourishment. Terrible sustenance is a more

checked the issue of young people in created nations.

 Up to 70,000 youngster in agricultural nations kick the bucket from confusions during pregnancy

every year. Youthful moms and their infants are likewise at more serious risk of contracting HIV.

The world health organization WHO

 appraises that the risk of death following pregnancy is two times as high if teens in the range of 15 and 19 years than for those between the periods of 20 years or more.

The maternal death rate can be multiple times higher for young ladies.

somewhere in the range of 10 and 14 than for ladies of around twenty years old.

Unlawful fetus removal moreover

holds many dangers for young ladies in

regions like sub-Saharan Africa.
 Takes a chance for difficulties are higher for young ladies 14 years or more youthful, in light of the fact that their pelvis has not yet grown completely; this might prompt issues with labor.
 Issues other than the age of the mother, for example, destitution and social help too influence the result. High school moms actually must can depend on the family and the
state to assist them with adapting, and instruct their youngsters. Young guardians who can depend on
family and local area support, social administrations and youngster care support are bound to
proceed with their schooling and land more lucrative positions as they progress with their
schooling.
 Being a youthful mother frequently

influences schooling. High schooler moms are bound to drop
out of secondary school. Ongoing examinations, however, have found that a considerable lot of these moms had currently exited school preceding becoming pregnant.

# SOLUTIONS

## 10 TIPS TO PREVENT TEENS PREGNANCY:

1. Be clear about your own sexual qualities and mentalities. It will be a lot simpler for you to converse with your kid in the event that you have thoroughly considered these inquiries:

What is your opinion about school matured teenagers being physically dynamic or becoming guardians

Who necessarily draws the sexual lines in a relationship and How could this be finished.

Is it true or not that you were physically dynamic as a high schooler and what is your opinion about that at this point. Is it true or not that you were physically dynamic before you were hitched and how do the solutions to these inquiries

influence what you will tell your kids?
What is your opinion about empowering adolescents to go without sex.
What is your take on adolescents utilizing contraceptives?

2. Chat with your kids early and frequently about sex and love.
Be explicit. The main thing you can do is to say the initial not many words. Tell the truth and be open.
 Listen cautiously to figure out what your kid as of now comprehends. Make your discussions this way and that two different ways. Consulting with your kids about sex won't urge them to turn out to be physically dynamic. Kids need the same amount of help understanding how connections work and the significance of 10 Hints for Guardians To Assist Their Youngsters With Staying Away from Adolescent Pregnancy sex as they do in

understanding how all the body parts work. What's the contrast between adoration and sex, tell your kids what you esteem and accept and afterward make certain to be a decent good example and walk the discussion.

your kid must feel open to asking you inquiries about anything, not simply inquiries regarding sex. Give your all to be an "askable"parent. Tell your kids that they can consult with you about anything they are thinking or agonizing over.

Kids say they need to examine these sorts of inquiries:

How would I realize I'm enamored.

Will sex carry me nearer to my sweetheart.

How might I know when I'm prepared for sex.

How might I know when I'm prepared to get hitched.

Will engaging in sexual relations make me more famous.

Will I be more adult and have the option to do more grown-up exercises.

How would I tell my better half/beau that I would rather not engage in sexual relations without losing him/her or harming his/her sentiments.

How would I answer when my better half/sweetheart constrains me to engage in sexual relationship and contraceptives, how would they function

Which are the most secure

Which work the best

Might you at any point get pregnant at the initial time

Be a parent with a perspective. These are the sorts of things you could tell your kid:

I think kids in secondary school are excessively youthful to have intercourses particularly given the dangers of Helps and other physically sent sicknesses.

Whenever you really do have intercourse, consistently use security against pregnancy and physically send sicknesses until you are prepared to have a kid.

In our family, we accept that sex ought to be an outflow of affection inside marriage. Youngsters today end up in many physically charged circumstances. Ponder how you will deal with this. Have an arrangement. Will you say no, Will you use contraceptives?

How might you haggle that it's regular and ordinary to have sexual cravings and to contemplate sex. It isn't acceptable for teenagers to get pregnant.

Having a child doesn't make a kid into a man or a young lady into a lady.

Individuals hold on until they are prepared to assume liability prior to having a youngster.

Having intercourse isn't the value you ought to pay for having a cozy relationship. Assuming it is, track down another beau/sweetheart

3. Administer and screen your kids' exercises.
Know where your kids are consistently. Could it be said that they are protected. What's happening with them Is it true or not that they are associated with helpful exercises in the event that they aren't with you, are dependable grown-ups administering them.
You might be blamed for being excessively snoopy, however you can assist your kids with understanding that guardians who care know where their children are.

4. Know your kids' companions and their families.
Since peers impact adolescents, put forth a valiant effort to assist your kids pick

companions from families with comparative qualities. Welcome your youngsters' companions into your home, and talk with them consistently. Talk with their folks about curfews, normal principles and assumptions.

5. Beat early, incessant and consistent dating down.
Empower bunch exercises. Well before your kid inquires as to whether the individual in question can date someone in particular, clarify that one-on-one dating before 16 can prompt difficulty. Telling your kids quite a bit early will assist them with seeing that you are not responding to a specific individual or greeting.

6. Take major areas of strength for and against teenagers dating individuals who are fundamentally more seasoned or more youthful than they are.

Take a stab at putting down a boundary of something like a 2 year age contrast. Power contrasts can lead into dangerous circumstances including undesirable and unprotected sex.

7. Assist your teenagers with having choices for the future that are substantially more alluring than early pregnancy and life as a parent. Assist them with setting genuine, significant objectives for their future. Talk with them about how they should arrive at their objectives, and assist them with arriving at these objectives. Assist them with perceiving how becoming a parent can crash the best of plans. For instance, youngster care costs can make it remarkably difficult to bear the cost of school.

Assist them with figuring out how to involve their extra energy in helpful ways, being certain they carved outside opportunities to get their work done. Local area administration can assist with showing them work abilities, and can place them in contact with different committed and caring grown-ups.

8. Accentuate the amount you esteem schooling.
Set exclusive requirements for your youngster's school execution. In the event that your kid isn't advancing great in school, mediate early. School disappointment is one of the key gamble factors for adolescent life as a parent. Monitor your kids' grades and meet with instructors. Volunteer at school if possible. Limit adolescent's after-school positions to something like 20 hours out of each week, so there is adequate time for schoolwork and enough time left over for peaceful rest and mingling.

9. Understand what your children are watching, perusing and paying attention to. Messages about sex sent by the media television, radio, motion pictures, music recordings, magazines, and Web are more than likely in conflict with your qualities. Be "media educated"about what you and your family are watching and perusing. Train your kids to think basically; talk with them about the things they are gaining from the projects they watch and the music they pay attention to.

Try not to permit TVs in your kids' rooms. You can likely not completely control what your kids see and hear, yet you can spread the word, and you have some control over what occurs in your home. Switch off the television, drop memberships, and be clear about what films, records and recordings are adequate.

10. Make progress toward a relationship

that is warm and loving, firm in discipline and wealthy in correspondence.

Stress common trust and regard.

Express your adoration, fondness and appreciation plainly and frequently.

Embrace your children and let them know the amount you love them consistently.

Listen cautiously to what your kids say.

Focus on what they do.

Spend fun, wonderful time with your kids everyday, if conceivable. This is the establishment for your relationship. It is the financial balance that will help you through the inescapable tough situations ahead.

Be caring and gracious to your kids, and let them in on you anticipate a similar consequently. Try not to look at one kid against another. Tell every kid he/she is stand-out and beyond value.

Assist them with dominating new abilities. Genuine confidence must be acquired as it was done in the good old days through having a decent outlook on what you do. Attempt to have somewhere around one family feast together every day. Utilize the time together to talk not to contend. Know that dealing with a decent connection with your child is rarely past the point of no return. Despite the fact that your adolescent might be behaving as she would rather not have at least something to do with you, those are most likely not her genuine sentiments. Offspring of any age need a cozy relationship with their folks, and they long for their folks' assistance, endorsement and backing.

# THE IMPACT OF TEENS PREGNANCY

Juvenile pregnancy stays a significant supporter of maternal and youngster mortality. Difficulties connecting with pregnancy and labor are the main source of death for young ladies matured 15-19 universally. Pregnant young ladies and teenagers additionally face other wellbeing dangers and inconveniences because of their juvenile bodies. Children brought into the world to more youthful moms are additionally at more serious gamble.

The impacts of teen pregnancies are numerous and unpleasant. Other than getting pregnant, the adolescent young ladies and their kids are in danger of being contaminated with sexually transmitted diseases including HIV/Helps. Also, there are wellbeing suggestions related to early sex and pregnancies like obstetric fistula, newborn child passing, maternal demise, eclampsia, and cervical disease. Furthermore, different intricacies happen because of the lacking pelvis of the young lady.

Additionally juvenile pregnancy can likewise affect young ladies, their families and networks. Unmarried pregnant youths might confront shame or dismissal by guardians and companions as well as dangers of brutality. Young ladies who become pregnant before age 18 are likewise bound to encounter savagery inside marriage.

Teen pregnancy likewise achieves physical and mental injury to the young lady since she is confronted with numerous problems presented to her by the family and

the general public. It additionally causes

the guardians to feel embarrassed in light of their supposed carelessness as seen by people in general or society.

**The impact of teens pregnancy are:**

- . **Family and Friend Backing:**
- . **Child**
- . **Training/Information**
- . **Mother.**

**Family and Friend Backing**

Teens moms can build their flexibility through having the help of their folks as well as keeping up with social relations with their friends. Having those associations all through your pregnancy and after as well as having all of that help enormously impacts the moms mentality and variation to her new job throughout everyday life. Besides, another defensive component which increments youngster mother versatility is in the event that the mother proceeds to move on from secondary school as opposed to exiting. The in general most significant variable is the adolescent mother having the help of her own mom. The mother of the youngster can be very useful as far as everyday reassurance for her girl as well as monetary guidance and assisting her girl with kid raising liabilities of the infant.

## Child

The child of a high schooler mother is

probably going to live in destitution in light of her moms absence of monetary assets. Basically, the introduction of this youngster turns into the start of a ceaseless cycle by and large. The kid is probably going to persevere through a large number of similar issues its mom did in her life as a youngster. For example, the youngster is probably going to experience childhood in destitution and in exceptionally unfortunate circumstances. They are probably going to be feeling the loss of a mentor, leaving them with less good examples and expanded possibilities of trusting in different youngsters experiencing the same thing. The kids' scholastic achievement is additionally compromised and these youngsters don't endeavor to accomplish much scholastically. Besides, these children have social issues and can't make companions effectively which prompts unfortunate relationship improvement which is a critical stage in pre-adulthood. Unfortunate relationship improvement can be connected to the kid being denied monetarily as well as instructively. The kids are probably going to exit secondary school and furthermore surrender to the utilization of medications and liquor because of absence of parental association and observing

The cycle is probably going to rehash the same thing again and again.

The youngsters are frequently additionally prone to endure well being and take a chance in contrast with those brought into the world by grown-ups. They are probably going to be intellectually debilitated and furthermore helpless to conduct issues.

The kids are probably going to be conceived underweight and rashly, which is adverse to their wellbeing and may try and bring about newborn child mortality.

# Training/Information

From early on, small kids and teenagers really should have a dependable and reliable grown-up to trust in. Having a congenial and learned good example or grown-up in your life will enormously diminish the possibilities of adolescent pregnancy. Guardians frequently disregard clarifying the life structures of the body for their kids, but giving this data and instructing youngsters during their childhood is a critical defensive element against adolescent pregnancy. Youngsters need to grow up having a positive mental self portrait as well as a sound climate to experience childhood in. Kids need unrestricted love and backing from their folks as it is basic in guaranteeing the kid goes with better decisions about their future sexual action.

Having love from one's folks guarantees that these teenagers are not left feeling undesirable from guardians who are exceptionally detached and uninvolved. Open correspondence and time enjoyed with kids is a defensive element against high schooler pregnancy moreover. Kids and youngsters ought to have the option to move toward their folks and request their time at whatever point out of luck. Fostering areas of strength for kids and parents is basic. These youngsters are bound to utilize anti-conception medication or different contraceptives and pursue better choices concerning sexual ways of behaving.

## Mother:

Because of becoming pregnant during youth, adolescent moms are probably going to exit school as a result of their low desires and devotion to getting training. Around 38% of female teenagers who have a youngster before the age of 18 complete their high school schooling by the age of 22. This implies that an extremely high level of youngster moms won't actually proceed to move on from secondary school, not to mention seek after post-optional instruction. Considering this, these little kids don't have full capabilities for legitimate positions from now on, which prompts having some work with exceptionally low wages or far more atrocious, joblessness. Further, this prompts unfortunate day to day environments and the powerlessness to keep a protected and clean climate for their infant youngsters. These young ladies frequently wind up living on government assistance and don't have sufficient assets for their kid. Generally, these little kids are compelled to defer and delay any designs for their future to bring up their kid.

One more issue related with high schooler pregnancy is the youthful mother is frequently compelled to surrender her character for another one while exchanging into a maternal job basically. These youthful moms go through numerous actual changes: from young adult actual acclimation to adjusting to the constantly changing state of her body through the pregnancy and her post pregnancy figure.

Youngsters are frequently compelled to become dependent on their family for monetary assets as well as to assist with helping her through bringing up a kid. Now and again, teenagers are disregarded by their folks and even get no help from their folks who are not tolerating the pregnancy.

These little kids are frequently compelled to lose contact with companions and others in their gatherings to zero in on their pregnancy.

Pregnant teenagers frequently don't have the legitimate sound propensities to go through a fruitful kid raising interaction. These moms consequently have uplifted wellbeing gambles, which represses sound youngster advancement. Young ladies can experience the ill effects of things, for example, weakness as well as circulatory strain which is just conceivable during pregnancy. These moms frequently smoke and drink since they are not as expected instructed on the youngster raising interaction.

Having a kid during these fundamental years genuinely conflicts with the formative errands that ought to happen during youths. These youthful moms can't completely foster an identity due to their new job as an anticipating mother. Further, companion and social connections are stressed or even ended and high schooler years are basically for creating associations with others and finding oneself Because of these variables, youngster moms might wind up creating melancholy after basically being estranged from their loved ones.

These side effects of melancholy increment the possibilities of the adolescent mother ending it all.

Chasing after this further, youngster moms are frequently stressed for assets and social help from the dad of the kid. At times, the youngster's father will stay present in the meantime and at others the dad will not.

In the event that the dad stays present there are many times high connections, strain and disappointment as a result of the absence of monetary assets, backing and kid care which will be required. There is an expansion in struggle which might prompt separations, passing on the mother to be a solitary parent or even brutality inside the relationship.

 Because of the absence of monetary assets, these young ladies frequently don't get pre-birth exams or normal tests for their child and accordingly they know nothing about any wellbeing worries for their kid.

A large number of these adolescent moms are not sufficiently beneficial, consequently they have a higher gamble for deterred work and furthermore these young ladies frequently go through dangerous fetus removals which lead to the demise of numerous youthful females and their unborn child.

Finally, young pregnancy has generally added to kid neediness, since the young ladies are compelled to exit school to deal with their children.

# PARENTAL CONTRIBUTION

well in school. Nonetheless, such cases frequently come from teens whose guardians are less associated with their scholarly exercises. The juvenile stage is a basic stage in an individual's life.

It is portrayed by extreme sentiments and feelings. Young people see their folks as either cool or unfeeling toward their sentiments. Continuous correspondence can assist guardians with building entrust with their kids. Hence, correspondence can be utilized as an instrument for surveying a youngster's sexual way of behaving, scholarly execution, confidence, and substance misuse conduct.

Certain individuals have the perspective that adolescent love is like different types of heartfelt love. They contend that it is human or normal to fall head over heels and in this manner, understudies ought not be denounced for taking part in heartfelt connections. Besides, figuring out how to cherish is a cycle that characterizes an individual's future relational connections. Teens accept that dating encounters set them up for adulthood relationship challenges. Notwithstanding, they neglect to consider the adverse results of adolescent connections, for example, high school pregnancies and STIs, which frequently cause heartfelt separations. Since youngsters are not ready to deal with relationship challenges, reasonable contentions frequently bring about heartfelt separations. Subsequently, the guardians' recommendation about dating can assist teens with figuring out the difficulties of connections and defer dating until they are prepared for it.

Precluding high school love can't tackle the issues connected with adolescent sentiment or deflect them from participating in sex. Hence, guardians can advance positive ways of behaving in their youngsters through sex training and directing. Also, guardians can act as good examples for their kids by persuading them to do well in school and offering them exhortation on the most proficient method to deal with youngster issues.

# THE CAUSES OF TEENS PREGNANCY.

One of the significant reasons for youngster pregnancy is nonattendance of tender management from guardians or gatekeepers. In the ongoing society, guardians are either excessively occupied or excessively lenient. Aside from the arrangement of essential requirements, guardians and gatekeepers are not engaged with close to home dependability of the young lady kid.
Teens, particularly young ladies, go through fascinating circumstances and changes in which they need parental help to comprehend and acknowledge the changes. On the off chance that they come up short on friendly management from their folks, they look for replies from sweethearts who appear to be offering the

love and consideration that winds up with a pregnancy.

One more significant reason for teen pregnancy is peer pressure. As youngsters develop to adolescent hood, there is expanded strain to squeeze into specific friend gatherings. The companions may then drive the young lady into having intercourse to fit well in their gathering. Furthermore, the cutting edge society permits the teens to have a great deal of existence with the other gender all alone, which results in cases of pregnancy at young age.

Different elements key to this idea is sexual maltreatment as well as the utilization of medications and liquor. Youngsters are presented to liquor and medications causing them to let go completely over their sexuality when tipsy along these lines prompting pregnancies. Sexual maltreatment then again happens when the young ladies go for sex for joy without figuring out the sexual effect. It is likewise obvious when a grown-up physically defrauds a young lady or a minor.

## What causes teen pregnancy.
. **Absence of data about sex.**
. **Low financial status.**
. **Absence of sex training in schools to young ladies.**
. **Media impact.**
. **Alcohol and drugs.**

**Absence of data about sexual and regenerative wellbeing and privileges**
Deficient admittance to administrations custom fitted to youngsters
Family, people group and prevailing burden to wed
Sexual viciousness
Youngster, early and constrained

marriage, which can be both a reason and an outcome
Absence of instruction or school drop-out.

## Low Financial Status

Adolescents who become pregnant frequently come from groups of low financial status. Growing up, these kids frequently come from families who are experiencing destitution and don't have every one of the essential assets to bring up their youngsters. These youngsters grow up to have low instructive objectives and triumphs in light of the absence of contribution from their own folks. These small children then, at that point, inclined toward a negative climate end up with less desire to prevail in school and start making fellowships with different teenagers who are going through comparative circumstances as them. These gatherings of adolescents start to explore different avenues regarding medications and liquor and don't do very well in school. additionally it is connected to low degrees of family connectedness. This implies that kids/youth experiencing childhood in these homes don't have major areas of strength for play models or people to gaze upward to or gain from. Inside these low financial status families, misuse is frequently predominant and inclines youth toward risky and upsetting circumstances. Whether the youngster is being mishandled or seeing homegrown maltreatment, youths are being isolated and disengaged from their families which could prompt unfortunate navigation. This absence of family connectedness drives youth away from trusting in the grown-ups inside their homes however towards other pained youth experiencing in the same

ways.
With their absence of training and information about propagation, these teenagers take part in unprotected and perilous sexual movement. These adolescents have close to zero familiarity with the accessible contraceptives nor do they investigate their choices. Regardless of whether the youths have some type of contraception they are utilizing them mistakenly which makes them futile during sexual action. These adolescents just participate in intercourse at exceptionally youthful ages, and may have various accomplices which further prompts expanded possibilities of pregnancy.

## Absence of sex training in schools to young ladies.

This has added additional expanded adolescent pregnancy. This is on the grounds that it prompts the liberal in sexual exercises without figuring out the potential impacts. It is hence critical to allow young ladies to comprehend issues encompassing sex and their sexuality as well as the potential effects.

This is the obligation of educators, strict guardians, and the whole society to confer the information. Then again, the media has added to adolescent pregnancy by promoting and showing programs, syndicated programs, as well as playing melodies that support sex. This makes teens practice what they see on the media accordingly winding up with pregnancies. Generally speaking, youngsters don't have the information on utilizing and getting to contraceptives, something that adds to high school pregnancies. Different factors, for example, financial and ecological issues are instrumental in causing adolescence.

# Media Impact

The media to a great extent affects youngster pregnancy, particularly shows, for example, High Schooler Mother. These shows frequently glamorize pregnancy and conceal the genuine difficulties related with pregnancy which urges these adolescents to become pregnant. A few young females become pregnant to make sure they can exit secondary everyday schedules and force their accomplices into a more profound responsibility. Resistance is likewise another justification for why a few teenagers will become pregnant. To show their freedom and consider themselves as having more command over their lives, a youngster might choose to have a kid. These TV series celebrate having a youngster through the advancement of these teens having a more grown-up way of life, with greater obligation and dynamic power.

## Alcohol and drugs.

During youthfulness, young people might drink and explore different avenues regarding drugs regularly with their companions at get-togethers and gatherings. Adolescents, nonetheless, don't understand the effects liquor and medications have on the working of their mind, particularly the impacts of hitting the bottle hard which is drinking a lot of liquor during one sitting. Drinking exorbitantly as well as testing medications might prompt undesirable and accidental pregnancy. These substances extraordinarily influence a youngsters capacity to coherently think and complete general reasoning cycles, hence expands the possibilities they will take part in unprotected and dangerous sexual action.

# THE GAMBLE (RISK) OF TEENS PREGNANCY:

The following are a couple of dangers that are more prominent on the off chance that you are pregnant before the age of 15 or you don't look for pre-birth care:
**low birth weight/untimely birth.**
**weakness low iron levels**
**hypertension/pregnancy-initiated hypertension**
**PIH can promp**t **toxemia**
Absence of pre-birth care.
Pregnant youngsters are in danger of not getting the right pre-birth care, particularly on the off chance that they don't have support from their folks. Pre-birth care is basic, particularly in the primary long

periods of pregnancy. Pre-birth care searches for clinical issues in both mother and child, screens the child's development, and manages any confusions that emerge. Albeit the high schooler pregnancy rate has declined by 55% beginning around 1990, teenagers are as yet becoming pregnant and conceiving an offspring and 75% of those are accidental pregnancies. While it is conceivable that a youngster who becomes pregnant can encounter a solid pregnancy and be an incredible parent, numerous pregnant and nurturing teenagers battle with various stressors, wellbeing gambles and other complex issues. Being pregnant as a teen puts you at a higher gamble for having a child conceived too soon, with a low birth weight and, unfortunately, higher gamble of death.

# What Are the Dangers

Assuming a pregnancy is impromptu, the mother may not be getting the pre-birth care she and her child need or may not actually be sufficiently solid to convey a youngster to term.

Adolescents are frequently caught off guard for the real factors associated with nurturing a newborn child. Frequently, complex connections and monetary weight joined with adjusting school and nurturing are distressing and can seriously endanger an infant.

Teenagers who are pregnant or raising a child struggle with completing school. Just 3% of youngsters who have a child accept their school certificate before the age of 30.

Numerous youngster guardians are single. Being a solitary parent can have monetary and close to home stressors and a focused on parent seriously endangers a child. Guardians frequently need assets to assist them with exploring their youngster's prosperity and improvement. Youngsters may not know about this sort of help.

How Can Be Diminished the Dangers.

Youngsters can forestall a pregnancy with powerful and simple conception prevention strategies that are generally accessible. Low-upkeep, minimal expense or free conception prevention are accessible at many specialist's workplaces and facilities. At Cross country Kids' Medical clinic, the Conception prevention for Teenagers Facility gives many kinds of anti-conception medication for young ladies up to the age or 25, including low support contraception, for example, an embed that is set in the upper arm and can forestall pregnancy for up to 3-10 years. Youngsters who test positive for pregnancy ought to know their choices and assets and act rapidly. Being pregnant can be close to home and terrifying for a youngster and she might be hesitant to tell her folks or a confided in grown-up. The Pregnancy Backing Guide, produced for pregnant youngsters, examines pregnancy choices, assets and answers often posed inquiries about pregnancy.

Youngsters who are pregnant ought to quickly shut down all utilization of medications, liquor or tobacco items. Moreover, they ought to eat a sound, adjusted diet and drink a lot of water.

On the off chance that the high schooler is going on with the pregnancy, she should plan a pre-birth care arrangement as quickly as time permits. The Adolescent and Pregnant Program at Cross Country Kids' gives pregnant young ladies (up to progress in years 21 ½), and their families, skilled pre-birth care, schooling and support to accomplish better birth results. TaP enables youthful, pregnant youngsters by giving them the instruments to have sound pregnancies, have solid children and be extraordinary guardians.

# YOUTHS SEX GUIDANCE (TEENS SEX EDUCATION)

Sex preparing for youths is the commitment of every parent and teacher. They can outfit adolescents with the right information so the last choices are not off course through various sources like magazines, friends, and destinations. As gatekeepers, countless us track down wrong and testing in any case the subject, and hence, this book is valuable. Right when your high schooler hits pubescence, a lot of changes can be figured out clearly, especially as for their body or facial hair development. These movements can be attempting to recognize, and consequently they go through a lot of mental episodes. Moreover, requesting that they stay away from explicit things that you could feel are denied constructs their tendency to explore them further. Consequently, give this book a read, and get the course you truly need to have an accomplished conversation with your high schooler.

Sex preparing fundamentals may be peddled in prosperity class. However, young people most likely will not hear or fathom all that they require to know to make hard decisions about sex. That is where you come in.

It might be wrong, but sex preparation is a parent's work. By interacting with your high schooler early and regularly, you can clear a path for an extensive stretch of sound sexuality.

# The following are a couple of considerations:

Make the most of the open door. Exactly when sex comes up in a show or tune, use it as a strategy for starting a conversation. Normal minutes like riding in the vehicle or dealing with food are commonly the best chances to talk.

Talk early and as often as possible. A one-time "sexual closeness"talk isn't adequate. Start bantering with your juvenile about safe sex during the young person years. Continue with the conversation into early adulthood. Change the conversation to suit advancement and improvement.

Come clean. If you're off-kilter, say exactly that. However, keep on talking. If you have no clue about how to answer your high schooler's requests, propose to find the reactions or think that they are together.

Be prompt. Clearly express your feelings about sex.

Give real factors about perils like near and dear anguish, truly conveyed pollution (STIs) and unconstrained pregnancy. Get a handle on that oral sex is certainly not a bet free choice instead of intercourse. Think about your young adult's point of view. Extreme conversations and scare procedures can stop affiliation and empower disobedient, dangerous approaches to acting. Taking everything into account, focus on your adolescent carefully. Sort out the pressures, hardships and stresses that teenagers have.

Move past current real factors. Your young person needs to acknowledge current real factors about sex. However, examining opinions, attitudes and values is equivalently huge. Young people will undoubtedly embrace family values when they understand their people and feel understood by them.

Revolve around thriving. The youth years are known as a time of chance taking. Be that as it may, then again they're while sound dealing with oneself approaches to acting beginning. Other than talking about risks, model and express the value of strong associations and choices.

Welcome more conversations. Tell your high schooler that it's okay to talk with you about sex when various types of criticism arise. Reward requests by saying, I'm cheerful you came to me.

Tending to hard subjects

Sex tutoring for adolescents integrates not having sex imitation date attack, direction character, sexual bearing and other hard focuses. Be ready for questions, for instance,

How should I understand I'm ready for sex? Many issues, for instance, peer strain, interest, and discouragement, could lead youngsters into early sexual development. Guarantee your juvenile that it's okay to hold on. Sex is an adult direct. Notwithstanding, there are substitute approaches to partner with someone. Get a handle on that comfortable conversations, long walks, fastening hands, focusing on music, moving, kissing, reaching and embracing are safeguarded approaches to sharing warmth.

Think about how conceivable it is that my assistant requirements to take part in sexual relations, but I don't. Be obvious that no reliably suggests no. Sex should never be constrained or obliged. Any kind of forced sex is attack, whether it's done by an outcast or someone your high schooler has been dating.

Raise to your adolescent that alcohol and meds can cripple social classes' decisions. Likewise, they can make people think less doubtlessly. Date attack and other unsafe conditions become more likely when alcohol and meds are involved.

Envision a situation in which I'm tending to whether I'm lesbian, gay, physically impartial, transgender or unusual. Various young people wonder about their sexual bearing, direction, character or explanation. Help your young person with understanding that youths are just beginning to research actual charm. These opinions could change over an extended time. Additionally, if they don't, that is fine. An unfriendly answer for your youth's sexual bearing, direct character or verbalization can have critical effects. LGBTQ youth have a higher rate of STIs, substance abuse, pity and tried implosion. Family affirmation can shield against these risks.

In particular, let your young person know that your love is unfit. Approval your juvenile for discussing their considerations.

Listen more than you talk.

**Unhealthy/Healthy Relationships.**
Dating brutality happens shockingly habitually. Around 1 out of 12 young people has nitty gritty going up against physical or sexual dating fierceness. So getting current real factors and dealing with them with your youngster is huge.
Alcohol or drug use
Keeping away from mates and social gatherings
Exonerating a dating associate's approach to acting
Acting scared around a dating accessory
Loss of interest in school or activities that were once fun
Questionable wounds, scratches or various injuries
Youths in hurtful associations have a higher bet of long stretch effects. These consolidate awful scores, raising a ruckus

around town hard and implosion tries. The near and dear impact of early unwanted associations may in like manner clear a path for future upset, unpleasant associations.

Consult with your young adult now about the meaning of strong associations. Model sound associations through how you partner with your high schooler and others. The delineations your juvenile advances today about respect, cutoff points, and understanding what is great and terrible will reach out into future associations.

Noting approach to acting

Expecting your juvenile is genuinely unique, it very well may be a higher need than at some other chance to move the conversation along. Whether or not you think your high schooler is ready, be open yet veritable in your technique. Remind your high schooler that you guess that sex and its liabilities ought to be seen in a serious manner.

Stress the meaning of safe sex.

Contraception. Guarantee your juvenile understands how to get and use contraception, for instance, condoms and origination counteraction.

Advance exclusivity.

A specific sexual relationship maintains trust and respect while cutting down the risk of STIs.

Put down reasonable places to pause.

Carry out curfews and rules about visits with colleagues. This is especially huge if you notice actual appeal between your juvenile and certain partners.

Your adolescent's clinical benefits provider can help also. A standard test can permit your high schooler the chance to examine sexual prosperity to simply the provider in private. The provider can help your adolescent with looking into contraception and safe sex. The provider can moreover help you with building your capacities to show your high schooler safe sex.

The provider may similarly pressure the meaning of routine human papillomavirus vaccination. This inoculation shields people of all sexual directions against genital moles and sicknesses of the cervix, backside, mouth and throat, and penis. People can generally get the inoculation between ages 9 and 26. Anyway, it is a portion of the time open for people more settled than age 26.

Looking forward

Your course is crucial to supporting your high schooler to become a genuinely careful adult. Come clean and talk from the heart. If your juvenile doesn't give off an impression of being enthusiastic about what you want to say with respect to sex, express it in any event. Your young adult is probably tuning in.

# BENEFIT AND INCONVENIENCE OF TEENS PREGNANCY:

It is crucial that the right assistance and services be available to help young parents navigate this difficult journey because teen pregnancy can have substantial and lasting effects on the lives of young parents and their children.

So there are inconveniences and also benefits of teen pregnancy, let's  look a 7 of  each of them.

## 7 BENEFITS AND INCONVENIENCES OF TEEN MOMS.

# BENEFITS OF TEEN PREGNANCY:

1. Early bonding with the child and forming strong parent-child relationships.
2. Increased sense of responsibility and maturity as they navigate parenthood.
3. Some young parents find motivation to excel in life and provide a better future for their child.
4. Learning valuable life lessons and developing problem-solving skills.
5. Potential support from family and friends to help with parenting.
6. A chance to break cycles of neglect or abuse through positive parenting.
7. Opportunities for personal growth and development through the parenting experience.

You may be nearer to your children, as

you are nearer in age

You start a family youthful, so you can do more things when you are not old, however are still inside the time of having children, and you can head off to college in your 30's as well, in the event that you can't go when your children are more youthful.

You will mend better after birth, since you are more youthful

You mature quick, this can likewise be something terrible

Will see more ages of family grow up

Energy levels will be higher

Can strengthen connections with child daddy/beau, guardians, companions.

Furthermore, I mean, you become a mother, and I wouldn't exchange that for anything.

# INCONVENIENCE OF TEEN PREGNANCY:

1. Higher risk of health complications for both the teen mother and the baby.
2. Limited educational and career opportunities due to the demands of parenting.
3. Financial strain and difficulties in providing for the child's needs.
4. Social stigma and judgment from peers and society.
5. Reduced time for personal growth and self-discovery during critical developmental stages.
6. Emotional and mental stress as they cope with the challenges of parenthood at a young age.
7. Possibility of strained relationships with family and friends due to unexpected

pregnancy.

Shuffling school, work, and your public activity is hard enough when you don't have a youngster, envision it with it.

It will probably be hard monetarily

ALL of your consideration goes to your children and you won't ever get alone time haha

Can destroy connections with child daddy/beau, guardians, companions and so forth.

Individuals will more likely than not be judgemental

Labor can be more enthusiastic, as your body/hips/pelvis may not be sufficiently grown.

Higher possibility of untimely birth, which is related to and can cause numerous medical conditions for the child.

Mature quickly can likewise be something to be thankful for.

It's important to note that teen pregnancy can have varying impacts on individuals, and support systems play a crucial role in helping young parents navigate these challenges

# CONCLUSION

Denying young relationships can't tackle the issues related with juvenile love. All things being equal, parental contribution in their youngsters' scholar and public activities can assist with lightning issues like teen pregnancy, STIs, fetus removal, and substance misuse. Instructing understudies about sex, connections, and contraceptives.

It can subsequently be said that teen pregnancy is an issue to the whole society. Also, since it is generally brought about by factors in the general public, it is the commitment of each and every individual from the general public including strict pioneers, guardians, educators, and the young people themselves to partake in resolving the issue.

# SUCCESS OMA

## A professional writer


At the point when I was nineteen years of age I was on a transport while heading to school where I was concentrating on a degree in Reporting and Media Correspondences.
I always come across teenage girls with pregnancy and what they are going through. From then I tell myself that there is a need to stop  teen pregnancy.

* 9 7 9 8 8 5 4 5 1 6 1 8 1 *